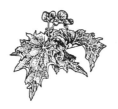

1997

Secret Waters

Linda C. Brown

Secret Waters

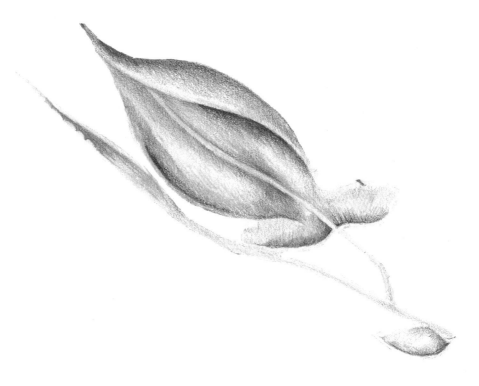

Blue Begonia Press • Yakima Washington

Acknowledgments

"Those Who Can, Do" was originally published by Blue Begonia Press in Wheel, a sHADOWmARK collection of broadsides.

This book was made possible, in part, by a grant from Artist Trust.

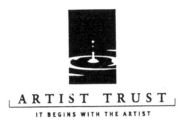

The colored pencil drawing, *Playing in the Shadows*, by Sue Grimshaw, was created especially for *Secret Waters*.

ISBN: 0-911287-24-8
Blue Begonia Press
225 S. 15th Ave.
Yakima, WA 98902-3821

Thanks

Thank you to both my parents. To my father who gave me stories and a sense of humor. To my mother who gave me a love of books and people. To my children, Seth and Paige, who think I'm funny as long as I "don't say that in public."

Thank you to the people who keep me sane. To John and Nancy Rossmeissl who have adopted me, warts and all. To Jane Schwab who refuses to let me rust. To Linda Pier who makes me laugh, even when we shouldn't. And to Bonnie Naasz for stories and joy.

A special thanks to all the caregivers at the Renaissance Care Center and those everywhere who take a job that can't be done and simply do it, every day, twenty-six hours a day, eight days a week.

And finally, thank you to all those who teach us every day by living out every moment with dignity and spirit.

This book is dedicated to Aunt Diane
who had the gift of love

CONTENTS

IV *Eventide*

I

"Just So"

"As long as one person remembers your name. . ."

"Just So"

Ten years ago my mother and I were comfortably living on different ends of the world. Each summer we endured a week's visit like a temporary case of the flu. Like many mothers and daughters, we loved each other, but we didn't particularly like each other. So, we gave each other 3,000 miles of breathing room. And it worked. Until Alzheimer's.

On August 8, 1993, the planets realigned. Mother was placed in a nursing home and my father came to live with me. That night as I sat in the dark, it would have been easier to believe that the sun now rotated around earth, than to accept that this darkest moment would become my greatest gift.

The daily journey into the tangled world of Alzheimer's and nursing homes, helped me find my mother. I discovered that each day we must laugh and love. That in each of us is a fearsome courage. That in our humanity is true dignity.

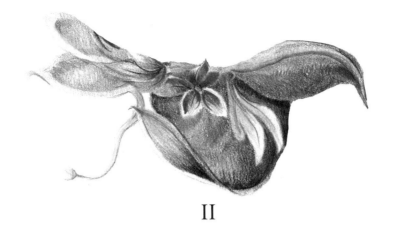

II

Ordering the Universe

"Wisdom has built her house. . ."

Proverbs 9

Beautiful Lady

The elevator door slides shut and we surge up five floors.
"Oooooh," Mother exclaims, a child on a carnival ride.
"What a beautiful lady!" I look to see where the voice is
coming from. Everyone in the elevator is smiling at Mother.
"Such a beautiful lady!"

I try to make myself look at her with this stranger's eyes.
Mother is a remarkably young 77. Her hair still golden. Her
make-up glows. She insists on rosy cheeks and spends hours
staring into a mirror, dusting them over and over with blush.
She is wearing lavender pants and matching sweater. Has worn
them every day this week. The style and color suit her, but I
cannot move beyond the torn hem or dark stains embedded on
the sleeves. She is, indeed, a beautiful lady, but I haven't a clue
who she is.

The Gardener

Mother grows plastic flowers. Stalks of extruded lilacs, straight backed and tall. Peonies, molded into fat flowering sea anemone. White lilies, stark and bare, fading in summer's harsh light. She arranges the pots on the kitchen table, turning their blooms toward a glaring sun. They flourish, each tenacious leaf a testimonial to her care.

"Your father never cared for flowers," she says. "Thought they were a waste of time. But I could always make things grow," she smiles. "It's a gift. The secret is knowing when to pinch back the old so tender new shoots can emerge." And she retreats to her garden, churning the soil, making this a place of beauty.

Dressed for Success

We often find Mother busily dressing at 3 a.m. and have long ago given up trying to show her the darkened sky. She tells us she is dressing for an occasion: a graduation party or a trip to the beauty parlor. Often these events are based in reality, but are days or weeks away. We try writing everything on a calendar. "Look," we show her. "Today is Tuesday and we have one-two-three days until your beauty parlor appointment on Friday." She nods with understanding, but when our attention shifts away she returns to her dress.

She wears three or four bras at the same time. Two or three blouses. She insists on wearing the same outfit repeatedly, impervious to the constraints of temperature and time: wool knit skirts and sweaters during the hottest week in July, high heels and necklaces for bed.

We dead bolt the closet doors, but in unattended moments mountains of clutter appear. June gives way to April and Wednesday follows spring.

Scavenger Hunt

Dad and I do most of the chores while Mother sleeps. It is easier that way. Besides laundry, I vacuum at night, while Dad tackles the kitchen. He keeps the dishwasher free from dirty dishes because Mother still sets the table. She uses dishes within eyesight, clean or not.

Her table settings vary. One day she puts out soup spoons. Another day, all knives. One night she circles the table with ten soup bowls. We no longer object. The activity boosts her spirits. It is better than those days when she forgets where the kitchen is and the names of familiar household objects.

Mother thinks the kitchen is her bedroom and shoes appear in the refrigerator and underwear in the dishwasher. We cannot turn on the oven without checking for foreign objects. Much of the food is now kept in a freezer under lock and key because packages of meat vanish until the stench of rotting beef leads us to the hiding place.

A House Divided

My visits disrupt Mother's world. I try to bring order to a house in turmoil. The changes confuse Mother. She imagines she is in a new house that Dad has built without telling her. "How did he do it?" she asks. "He has built a house almost exactly like ours only not as nice." Agitated, she demands to be taken back to "my house." Just when we hope this has passed, it surfaces again and we must contend with her insistence that she will not stay in this strange house for even a second longer.

Arguing is pointless. And trying to imagine how her mind is functioning is equally futile. The only success we have is playing along and diverting her attention. We manage getting her to return to bed telling her we're afraid to drive home in the dark. "Tomorrow," we say, "home will be easier to find."

The Betrayal

My father and I sit like expectant parents at the geriatric center. Mother plays with her handbag examining coupons for Rice-A-Roni and cream pies. She reads aloud to no one in particular.

She's worse, my father says to the case worker, eyes apologizing for this betrayal. But we can manage. Yes. She knows me. And, of course, Linda, our daughter. Most of the time. Most of the time.

Across the expansive desk lie answers, but we dare not ask the questions. If we know more, we will drown.

Mother takes a battery of tests. The questions play in our minds as though the answers are the key to sanity. Always there is the doubt: who are the sane? Can she name five presidents of the United States? Of course, she can. There's Roosevelt. He's the President now, isn't he? Can she remember the following concrete items: chair, table, lion, orange, and rose? How silly, she says, but can recall none. When prompted that one is a fruit, she brightens. I remember now. A pineapple!

My father studies his hat in disbelief. "Annette," he sighs, "you don't even like Roosevelt!"

The Decision

Mother attends a day camp twice a week. A van picks her up and we wave her away each morning hoping she'll remember us on her return. She comes home full of chatter and cupcakes. Each day another birthday. While she is at play, Dad and I drive to nursing homes, but never go in.

The phone rarely rings. Mother busies herself with visits from the characters on *The Young and The Restless*. Dad does his books, adding, subtracting, adding again. Nothing ever in balance.

When the time finally comes, Dad's conviction fails. "I promised her I would never put her in a nursing home," he says. "I can't break that promise. I won't!"

Mother happily waters a plastic flower arrangement. A river forms, cascading off the kitchen table and onto the floor. "I gave her my word," he repeats. "You do it!"

And the matter is settled.

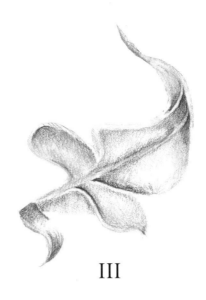

III

Gathering in the Moonlight

". . .she has also set her table."

Proverbs 9

The Comings and Goings

Connie, who sounds like a train conductor, sits at the front entrance bellowing out the comings and goings of visitors as they try to slip quietly into and out of the nursing home. Each pauses to catch a breath as the too familiar smell of disinfectant mingles with the smell of urine and aging flesh. "Here's the lady," she sings. "Here's the lady. She's coming. Coming. Here she is."

The visitor smiles trying to slip past a gauntlet of wheelchairs.

The basso profundo voice calls out departures as well. "Where are you going?" she calls, punching the "where" on her first call. The emphasis shifts as she rolls down the sentence. "Where are you going?" she calls. Going?

Anxious leaving. Promising sky. Just beyond locked doors. A code of numbers, a sequence to follow—easy for those who do not live here. Hurry. The conductor's voice grows. Hurry. Try to remember. The train is coming.

Nailing the Moment

Ladies Beauty Club meets every Tuesday. The ladies clothed in sweat suits or housecoats roll into the dining room. They extend arthritic hands, supplicant cups ready to receive absolution or a candy bar. Three young girls dive into the task of manicuring each one in colors like Fire and Ice or Maui Sunset or Pomegranate and Roses.

Now they sit, a Greek chorus lining the hallway. Sarah, her black hair, never situated quite on the top of her head, bangs lapping down touching black eye glasses. Melda, shrunken so small, she looks like a head and legs in the huge gerry chair. Dora, this month's Resident of the Month, came to Yakima in 1918 from Iowa. And, of course, Aurelia, whose sharp nose and sharper eyes stand watch over the lot.

There they sit—a wreckage of womankind in a row, hands fluttering as they talk—looking every bit like finely feathered birds—sparks of reds and pinks and rose punctuating each tale.

Evening Vespers

Geneva walks the open corridor of the Renaissance Care Center. Her bobbed head bent low as if searching for loose change on the polished linoleum or studying the marbled pattern that stretches into endless turns and niches.

Each day she whispers past the chorus of ladies in wheel chairs lined up outside the now quiet dining room. Shuffling in cloth slippers, her feet never quite leave the floor. A smile touches her lips. Her eyes never lift from the path. She follows a road within her.

Shuffling the length of the corridor, soundlessly, gently, she turns east where the hallway bulletin board announces the Resident of the Month. This month is Melda. Several photos of Melda as a young woman stare down from the board decorated with orange and black crepe paper that carries out a Halloween theme.

In rituals there must be no hesitation. She doesn't miss a step toward her destination. The new fish tank in the parlor just at the end of the next hallway.

Head bowed she continues undaunted by the medicine cart blocking the hall. A voice calls for help. "For the love of Jesus, somebody. . .!" A bed pan pounds on metal railings in a nearby room. Geneva moves steadily, undeterred.

The Aquarium

They swim in a choreographed water ballet: neon tetras, guppies, mollies black as shining nights, angelfish. Darting lights weave between small mountains of red coral, plants bob in tropical waters.

But it is the miniature sharks that we study. They swim upside down, bellies turned skyward. We watch them, waiting for them to dive or leap or raise a fin in protest. We worry about them as though Esther Williams and Burt Lancaster have forgotten to breathe.

The experts at the local pet shop tell us that the fish are in shock and that they soon will die. Death is something we understand and so each day we look for telltale signs. But, the two crazy sharks continue to swim in a world gone topsy-turvy.

The residents keep watch. Bobbing and weaving, they roll past the tank on silent wheels. They study the tiny fish darting inside this beautiful glass prison. But it is the sharks they come to see. The crazy sharks swimming upside down, refusing to die.

Night Shift

I have lost the name of the nurse who works at the home, but would rather sell real estate. Roberta, I think. She brings laughter and humor to the job. She says she loves all these crazy people. Would love them even more if she could just get out of this crazy place. "Look at this wonderful face," she says, cupping the chin of a woman who smiles with the face of a ferret. Her whiskers stiff as a stranger's kiss.

"Look at this wonderful face," she laughs. "If I move that little house on Hillside," she whispers, "I'm out of here. History." And she glides down the hall calling to each patient she passes, "Honey, you're sure looking good today. Ain't it the truth. Ain't it the truth!" Her laughter causing little earthquakes as she goes.

Nursing the Hurt

There are a dozen faceless nurses. White blurs, that fly silently like shuttlecocks in and out of patients' rooms. Hummingbirds at the lily's cup. They glide smoothly through the stench of Lysol and urine. Through a choking chorus of complaints. Their demeanor never alters. Not even when Lena falls from her gerry chair and hits the floor like a porcelain teacup. Not even when Rob throws a dish against the wall watching the stain form a dark moon.

The nurses have a schedule to keep. Checking watches, they move quickly. Precious time. Time for meds. Blood pressures. Stool softeners. Time. Time. Spongy shoes squeak a cadence as they move with precision through time.

Zen Talk

"Time is time," Mother says. For a moment she has a look of her old self. I nod my head. Yes. Time is time. "Time is the matter," she says and for the first time in months we're having ourselves an old-fashioned conversation, a dialogue, an exchange.

"Shoes are the matter," she says and this, too, is good, because she is staring at my feet. I am wearing sandals which she cannot stand. This goes back to the beginning of time, her dislike of feet, and now we are both staring at my fat, chubby, albeit cutish, toes. "You hate my sandals, right?" I ask. And she laughs like we've shared a joke.

"Chairs are the matter," she says. We are moving to some new level of communication, reaching, trying to find connections between time and shoes and chairs.

Being Reduced to the Right Size

Dad is too sick to visit Mother, so I go alone. She sits quietly in her gerry chair—alone in her room. Quiet seems unbelievable in this place of too many people. I have brought her French fries which for once is the right thing to have done. She sucks on each, a bird extracting worms.

Vacant eyes wander the room, landing on me. "You look wide," she says and I am twelve years old again. I have broken her first rule of fashion: a short person wearing wrong way stripes.

"Is Dad doing something with Steve?" she asks. Amazing. Two coherent sentences in eight months and each one cuts me off at the knees. In one, I am fat. The other resurrects an ex-husband. Ten years blown away like dust.

As I clear away the few remnants of French fries, Mother vanishes into the hall, a river of linoleum. By the time I reach the door, she is walking away, arm in arm with Pete in his farmer's overalls. American Gothic. They move off toward a bank of wheel chairs, into the setting fluorescent lights.

The visit apparently over, I kick myself for having eaten too many fries. She's right. I look wide in this shirt. The stripes go the wrong way.

Unraveling Alzheimer's

Mother searches the corridors looking for a familiar face or a shiny bauble. Her eyes are vacant like film from which the images have faded. She wanders the halls halted only by the nice man's visits.

Eight months in the Renaissance Care Center (please, don't call it a nursing home), and Mother's hair has grayed. Her broad shoulders stoop and her walk has become a shuffle. When I watch her coming my way, I wonder who plays in the playground of her mind. I always believed that each moment serves a purpose, only now, I, too, search for meaning. I watch this once strong woman unravel as though someone holds a loose thread from her sweater and as she moves away it comes undone, stitch by pearly stitch.

Brides Wear White

"I'm getting married," she says. Only it's tough to understand because she has lost one plate of her dentures for sure and the other plate has been misplaced, to use the social worker's term. "It'll turn up," she says. "They always do," she smiles. "Either it's buried in a pocket of her clothing or maybe she left them in somebody else's room. But they'll show up." And she smiles again, a toothy grin.

I do not mention that the upper plate has not shown up since last September and that I've given up hoping to see them in someone else's mother's mouth. Besides, my mother has just announced her engagement and I'm a bit disconcerted, but not as disconcerted as my father, her husband of 59 years.

"He's very handsome," she says. But it comes out sounding more like, "Hiss vewy hissome." Why are you dressed like that?" she says to the nurse who fills the doorway. "The bride wears white," mother exclaims. Only it slides out of her mouth as "De bwide wes why." This tickles me except that she crumples onto the bed sobbing and I am struck by how red her face has become and how this could spoil an otherwise lovely wedding day.

"If this don't beat all," my father says shaking his head. "Now I've heard it all. She's marrying someone else," he says, and once again shakes his head as though ridding himself of the moment.

Rob

Rob rides the hallways. Strange man. One ear protrudes like a sail and the other clings to the side of his head. "I'm blind," he says, but I can't be sure. His eyes seem to wander like a floating compass, but sometimes they focus or at least fix on some image. What tickles me is the way he moves his wheel chair, his legs crossed at the ankles. He tiptoes forward like a sneaky ballerina.

Mother likes to care for Rob. "Now, Rob, look what you've gone and done in your pants," she'll say. And he looks down at the spreading circle of dark blue. Then, I remember he's blind. Maybe what he sees is mother's voice scolding him like a child, fussing over him, senselessly clucking, and he pirouettes in his chair, tiptoes off, his head tilting and shifting from side to side. Perhaps catching the wind.

Agnes

Mother is afraid of Agnes. Everyone is afraid of Agnes. If she weren't riding in a wheel chair, you'd swear that she walks with a swagger. Agnes doesn't take any "guff". That's what the head nurse calls it. "Stay out of Agnes' way, because she doesn't take any guff!"

Agnes comes rolling down the hall decked out in bedroom slippers with feathers and wearing a mile and a half of plastic beads. "I'll call 1-1-1." she says with menace in her voice. "That's just what I'll do, you crazy bitch. I'll call 1-1-1. Get you arrested!!" She seems to be speaking to no one in particular. Her voice has conviction.

I want to ask why she is so angry, but there's no sense messing with Agnes. She rolls down the hallway, twirling plastic beads like a lasso. At the end of the hall she pauses to accost a nurse. "Out of my way, bitch," she says, flashing a big grin, twisting her pearls.

Walking Away

Ted doesn't belong in the nursing home. He's a temporary. Came there just to recover from his leg that they had to lop off just below the knee. "Diabetes," he says, "but soon's it's all healed, I'm outta this place." He's been here since September watching the wound heal and harden. "Has to be tough enough to handle the leg they make me. But, when I've got my new limb, I'm getting up outta this chair and walking out," he says and hits a callused fist on the arm of his wheel chair to punctuate the sentence.

In January, Ted says, "I'm getting pretty close to breaking outta this place. Soon as my new leg gets fitted I'm a free man." But the snows come and it is too dangerous to try the leg outside. Inside too many people wander the halls, so he can never learn to maneuver.

By March, Ted seems a bit depressed. The leg has worn a sore spot on his stump and needs to be refitted. Once again he roams the corridors in a wheel chair—one leg buried in a cowboy boot, the other bobbing like a masthead on a boat.

In June, Ted gets the new prosthesis. It's the news of the day. "See you got your new piece!" or "How's the game leg?" Several of the ladies ask about his "prosthetic" only it sounds sexual the way they say it.

Ted rides the hallways with both legs deep in cowboy boots and saying good-bye to everyone. "Won't be long now." Only an infection sets in. Some think it's 'cause of the summer heat.

The Social Director

The social director's an old fashioned girl—always dressed in floral prints that swing like shifting flower gardens as she walks. She plans activities every day to help the patients pass the time, so they forget that they're here in the elephant burial ground and that Death is their fourth for bridge.

Today is movie day. A new Cary Grant film or Donald O'Connor and *Francis the Talking Mule*. They've seen *Mary Poppins* three times and *Sound of Music* twice, but no one remembers or cares.

What they need is a good film with sex and violence. Maybe a few viewings of *9 1/2 Weeks* will get pacemakers moving. A few shots of Kim Baisinger smearing her breasts with strawberries and cream will awaken dulling appetites and help digestion. That's the answer.

Cancel the Thursday Bingo session and Wednesday night's ice cream social. Call off Tuesday's pet day. Put the social director in a gold lamé dress with a plunging neckline and let her serve up Mickey Rourke and Kim sliding through the secret whispers of lust.

Now that's an activity worth dying for.

Table Talk

The annual hearing on Mother is slated for the twenty-fourth of August. Family members are invited to participate. Dad says he knows all he needs to know. "She's sick," he says. "What else can they say?" But I have questions that need answers.

The staff gathers around a conference table. The meeting is brisk. The language distant: cyanotic fingernails, inappropriate sexual advances, weepy and emotional, losing the ability to walk, does not transfer independently. Like tossing a hot coal around the table: Item 501 is linguistics, 502 is psychological, 503 is liquid intake, 504 is. . .

Suddenly the meeting ends. The head nurse speaks in the past tense. "It was good of you to come." She pushes back her chair to stand, but I am the only one who will be leaving. My questions have not been voiced. They will keep. The next meeting will be in February.

At home dad asks, "What did they say?" I glance at my list and tell him, "She's sick."

Simon Says

The new activities director, Frances, makes clever bulletin boards that say things like "Purrrrr-fect People" with photos of residents pasted in cats' heads. Frances replaces Leah, the redheaded one who went to Paradise, another nursing home. How would you like to be an elderly person and be told that soon you'll be in Paradise?

Frances says she'll be around a long time. She likes working with Leo, the guy with the pony tail who replaced Louis. Lou took a job at Del Monte sorting peaches or was that Ruben, the one who wore gold chains and hummed off key.

The residents need to go outside now that the weather has turned, Frances says. John, the new maintenance guy, promises to finish the garden courtyard. Last year, Marty planned to, but got sidetracked.

When John finishes, Evelyn, the cook who took over Myra's shift, will plant tomatoes. It won't take long for Joe to weed the flower beds. Of course, not right now, because this month he's working a double shift.

Frances takes a breath and waves like she's performing with a couple of hand puppets. She needs to move along. They're a little short-handed today.

Bearing Witness to Minor Miracles

Each morning Chip arrives before sunrise in the red Dodge truck that his only son got for him. He packs a thermos of black coffee and an undaunted smile. At dinner he fills in the gaps of the nursing home routine chatting about new arrivals and those who have found the "gentle death". Marie holds Chip's hand and like a young robin swallows his words.

Homesteaders from Hayden Lake. Survivors of the depression. They still live by the watchwords of Smiley Burnette on the radio, "Eat it up. Wear it out. Make it new." Sometimes they grew beans and carrots. Sometimes, a garden of stones.

"We had everything a person could want," Chip says. "We had a few cows and pigs. Fresh eggs every day and on Saturdays I'd get us a chicken and Marie would cook it up for Sunday dinner. Even had us a few horses." He speaks to Bernie and Lena and me, but his eyes belong only to Marie. They had very little, but they had it all.

"Is this the way to Willow Lane?" Lena asks of anyone who passes, hoping for the kindness of strangers. But no one seems to know the way and she is left with the cartography of glossy linoleum. Each hall takes her further from the promise of home.

She wanders the halls stopping at each crosswalk to look down the corridors. She hesitates, searching for familiar landmarks, then pushes forward. Her hand travels the highways of banisters and doorways. She has come a long, long way.

"Is this the way to Willow Lane?" she asks and each time the answer fails her she travels new byways until an opportunity to ask again. "Is this the way to Willow Lane?" "Yes, it is. Just around that turn." And she brightens. "I thought so," she says. "I thought so."

Those Who Can, Do

The woman next door to mother sits naked in her gerry chair. Two sagging breasts fold within crossed arms. A turban covers thinning hair and eyes visit some other place—far away.

"She walked as naked as could be," Dad says, "not wearing so much as a handkerchief. Down the hall to the nurses' station and back." His voice doesn't blink. I try to imagine my proper dad, bred with silver spoons and British upper lips, studying the woman's figure as she walks the 100 yards away and returns. I know he was smiling almost to the point of laughter.

"She used to be a school teacher," he tells me later as though I should have seen our kindred spirits. As though an admonition: this could happen to you. Will happen to you. And I laugh trying to imagine me years from now. No longer standing naked before students, but cursed with the final nursing home walk. I'd like to think that I would at least be carrying a book. Just the prop to add a sense of dignity. No, I quickly amend the vision. A scarlet rose. That will get people's tongues to wagging.

Messing Around

I am shopping for diapers again. They line the shelves of Safeway where aspirin and toothpaste and hemorrhoid ointments live. Long shelves of huge packages of products with titles that sound like sensitivity groups: Depends, Attends. They are covered in bright packaging like a party's inside. But the only party is that your mother or father or Aunt Sarah or Uncle Rob has taken to wetting herself or making a mess.

The language of babies is back, too. Mom shifts from foot to foot like she's got an itch way down deep and you say stupid things like, "Are you messing in your pants?" And she looks at you like you're crazy, because if she understood a stupid phrase like "messing in your pants", she wouldn't be doing it.

Mother's Day

The nursing home is closed down. A croupy cough has been taking a toll on the residents. Mother sits in isolation, locked in her gerry chair. Nothing to occupy her mind. No mind to occupy.

"It's Mother's Day," I tell her. "I've brought you flowers."

She stares at me with empty eyes and says, "Doo ti doo do do," which is her way of communicating now. She sings small songs that are her songs. They belong to her only. Sometimes they are sad and sometimes happy and sometimes it is hard to know because the words are always the same, "Doo ti doo do do."

When my friend Jane's mother was dying, she also seemed to lose her words. In her final days, she was left with only three: "I love you." And she'd repeat them in a low guttural voice filled with centuries of love behind them. "I love you."

A person can do something with "I love you". What's a person to do with "Doo ti doo do do?"

Later, as I am leaving the nursing home, the village ladies in the front hall chime out, "Happy Mother's Day". Happy, indeed. And without a thought I wave and sing, "Doo ti doo do too."

Marge

Nurse Marge has swallowed the moon, so when she moves down the corridor at the Care Center she radiates light. She moves fast and deliberately. She sweeps up the patients like gathering pieces of moonlight, because she owns the sky.

Some fear Marge's size and force. What do they know of lunar eclipses? What do they know of tide pools or moonlight?

My dad calls Marge "The Fat One." He has to be taught about the moon's constancy. With practice he has learned that she is "You know, the round one, Marge." She lifts mother like flower petals and drops her lightly where she can watch the ebb and flow of the nursing home. Mother loves the moon and I watch her give herself over to the light.

IV

Eventide

"Stolen water is sweet,
and bread eaten in secret. . ."

Proverbs 9

Farmer Pete

"That guy at the Renaissance Care Center died," Dad says. He has taken to reading the obituaries. Everyone listed in this week's paper has been in his 70's. Dad is 85. Actually, 85 last month. Now, he tells people that he's almost 86.

"Pete," he says again. "The one in overalls."

I look at the paper that he's still holding. "Dad, this guy's name is Horace." "But, look," he says, pointing. "This man died at the Renaissance Care Center. It has to be the same man. See, it says he is a farmer. And Pete is a farmer."

"How did you learn so much about this man? How do you know he's a farmer?"

"Overalls!" he says, disgusted at my stupidity. "He wears overalls, doesn't he?"

Later, at the center, we see Pete at his usual command post at the front window. One hand is buried deep behind the bib front on his overalls. The other hand waves across the window's expanse like a conductor with a baton. We never speak of him again.

The next day Dad looks up from his reading, "This town is a dangerous place to live. Even 60-year-olds are dropping like flies."

Feeding

We are filling up the ship with food for the hungry, overseas. A child in Belgium will go to bed with a full belly of whipped potatoes. The French are getting pureed beans and Jell-O. The British, well, food has never been too important to them. Tonight we are feeling generous, Mother and I. We send the Brits a cup of tea and giggle at the idea of tea going to England.

We've got our own little Marshall Plan going here. Some foods are airlifted in helicopters of silver spoons. Others swing on board in huge nets held high by human derricks.

This is the mother load setting sail with a cargo of tapioca. Only the ship is listing in the harbor. We can never load enough. No matter how much we send there will still be a hunger.

Letting Go

The school teacher is dying. She doesn't pull the mattress off her bed any more and it's been over two weeks since she walked naked down the long corridor to the nurses' station. The nurses think she's finally adjusted to nursing home life. But that's not possible. How can anyone get used to the lie in the shining linoleum floors or the shrill night cries.

No. They're wrong. The school teacher is dying. Otherwise she'd be throwing lime sherbet against the walls or stealing the photos of Jesus that adorn every dresser. She'd be pulling the fire alarm again to see how long it takes to lock down the building. She'd be plugging toilets with huge rolls of toilet paper creating lakes of water on the otherwise placid linoleum.

She's slipping away. She no longer covers her thinning hair with a Greta Garbo turban. She no longer demands gin and tonics with dinner. The fire is gone from her eyes. She's given up. Letting go. Dying. Just like us all.

Bernie

The women steal glances at Bernie, the handsome man in room 46. The men gossip about his age. "To look so young!" they say in hushed tones, combing tortured fingers through thinning hair. But Bernie's body is an unfaithful mistress. He cannot speak or swallow. Words forming in his mind lie stillborn.

He measures the world in diminishing increments, hungering for a way to breach the silence. Occasionally he communicates with the help of a spelling board. One young nurse tucks a pillow behind his back and he offers her a sacrament delivered one letter at a time. "y-o-u-h-a-v-e-b-e. . ." but she is gone before he can tell her of the beauty of her eyes.

At night I dream of the handsome man in room 46. He emerges from his chrysalis and we dance into the night. And each time he whispers a word, it becomes a new star in the galaxy lighting up the winter sky.

The Hat

Bill comes every day quiet and steady as the seasons. He stands just outside the door. There in the space where the world divides into two hemispheres. Susie has been here for six months. Six lifetimes. She marks the days by his shadow in the doorway. Bill is here. It is day. Bill is not. It is night.

He stands now in gray trench coat, brown felt hat. He fingers his hat, the way men do, circling the brim with a sweep of his hand, pinching the lid, caressing it in his hands.

He enters the room, her Humphrey Bogart. She, his Lauren Bacall. No words are needed. It's a new day. They have won again. He places the hat gently on a nearby chair, touches her hand. Death hasn't a chance in this scene.

Nearby, Mrs. Ramsey, lies in her bed, trying to become invisible. She's an extra in this intimate scene. She fumbles with a glass of water. Adjusts the volume on the t.v. Pretends sleep. The tension is palpable.

Finally, she can stand the silence no more and sighs the way old wooden bridges sigh under unfamiliar weight. "Excuse me," she says. "That's the most well behaved dog I've ever seen."

The lovers look at each other. Then at Mrs. Ramsey. But, she is smiling. Waving. Teasing the well behaved brown hat sitting on the chair.

Mae

The new woman at Mother's table has a broken heart. It is always hard for the new ones. They are still connected to the world beyond the curtains. New ones still try to control their world. The room is too hot. Too cold. I can't eat dairy. Pork chops are disagreeable. No salt on the table.

Mae likes potatoes. Each night she asks the most important question in her universe. "Can I have mashed potatoes?" The aides scurry, hoping to please, to appease. Tonight? Yes.

Tomorrow she will ask again. Mashed potatoes? Again the answer will be yes. It is always yes until she no longer asks.

Those who know have an unspoken agreement. They say "yes" to the world. It is easier that way. Hungry? Yes. Did the medicine help? Yes. Ready to return to your room? Yes. Glad to be alive? Yes.

But Mae is new. She does not understand. "Are you well tonight, Mae?" She shakes her head. "No," she says. "I am not well at all. Not at all."

Behold the Night

The polished floors are disquieting. My footsteps reverberate and the world seems hollow and empty like visiting a home where no one lives. Mother rests in bed exploring the swells and valleys of her body. Too absorbed in her own geography to know that I am there. I watch her for a while wondering if you ever get use to losing someone you don't even know. Then ease out of this place of strangers.

Down the hall, Bernie lies in silence, his back turned toward the door. I watch his shoulders rise and fall, listen to the labored breaths, the rattle of bones. Lena, too, is asleep, curled tight and small beneath a floral quilt. The whole facility holds a dreadful stillness.

I reel from the weight of not belonging. And celebrate it, too. Pulling my coat more tightly around me, I step out into the night. An icy wind gathers in the west. Each sharp breath clears away recent memory. The parking lot is almost empty. Chip is leaning against the tailgate of his truck. When he finally notices me, it is too late for either of us to pretend. His pain rises in clouds, "I love her so much," he says. "You know, most of the time I don't even know who she is." And we hold each other, this stranger and I, because of the cold.

The Stars

Patients come and go too fast. With every turn of the stile the pattern in the kaleidoscope shifts. New faces every day. The dining room is full of brittle fragments. Shards of broken colors that move from table to table like a carnival or a parade.

Scraps of people who have no names. Nameless stars in our firmament. Like a still sky refracted against secret waters. And so we name them: Orion and Leo, Cassiopeia and Ursa, Plowman and Swan. This is how we keep them alive. We never say good-bye to stars. Our constellations.

About the Author

Linda C. Brown was born and raised in Atlanta, Georgia to a family whose greatest gift was laughter. She studied at The Woman's College of the University of North Carolina and graduated from Ohio State University.

Linda lives in Yakima, Washington with Jack Clein, her father. They share their home with a golden retriever named Murphy Brown, and Felix, a cat with an attitude. Linda has two children, Seth and Paige, and thousands on loan for the school season, where she has taught English at A. C. Davis High School for more than twenty years.

Secret Waters is her first book.

About the Artist

Sue Grimshaw teaches art at A. C. Davis High School in Yakima, Washington. She shares her life with her husband, Dean, and her three cats and two Bassetts.

She incorporates pieces of life, emotional imagery, and cultural symbols, in drawing, painting, jewelry and fiber arts. Her colored pencil drawing, *Playing in the Shadows*, reflects the energy and spirit involved in the labor intensive layering of colors.

Grimshaw's art work has been shown throughout the Northwest; and she has been represented in, and won, numerous awards in juried competitions. She enjoys doing commissioned art projects such as the one she created for the cover of this book.